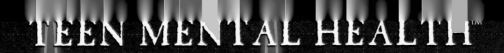

TEEN MENTAL HEALTH™

bipolar disorder

Jennifer Landau

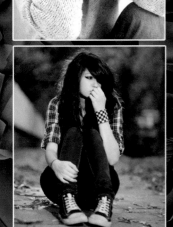

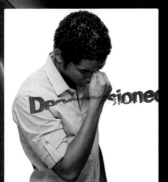

ROSEN
PUBLISHING®

New York

Published in 2014 by The Rosen Publishing Group, Inc.
29 East 21st Street, New York, NY 10010

First Edition

Library of Congress Cataloging-in-Publication Data

Landau, Jennifer, 1961–
Bipolar disorder/Jennifer Landau. — First edition.
    pages cm — (Teen mental health)
Includes bibliographical references and index.
ISBN 978-1-4777-1747-9 (library binding)
1. Manic-depressive illness—Juvenile literature.
2. Manic-depressive illness—Treatment—Juvenile literature.
3. Teenagers—Mental health—Juvenile literature. I. Title.
RC516.L36 2014
616.89'5—dc23
                                    2013013848

Manufactured in the United States of America

CPSIA Compliance Information: Batch #W14YA: For further information, contact Rosen Publishing, New
York, New York, at 1-800-237-9932.

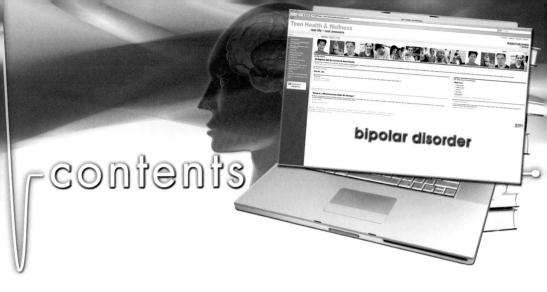

bipolar disorder

contents

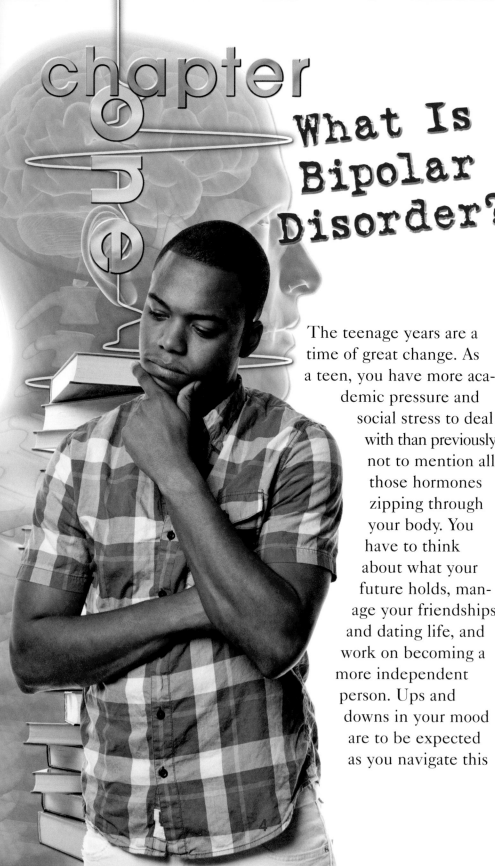

chapter one

What Is Bipolar Disorder?

The teenage years are a time of great change. As a teen, you have more academic pressure and social stress to deal with than previously, not to mention all those hormones zipping through your body. You have to think about what your future holds, manage your friendships and dating life, and work on becoming a more independent person. Ups and downs in your mood are to be expected as you navigate this challenging part of your life.

Bipolar disorder—what used to be called manic depression—is something different. According to the National Institute of Mental Health (NIMH), bipolar disorder is a "brain disorder that causes unusual shifts in mood and energy." This change is not teenage moodiness, but *extreme* shifts between mania and depression, the two poles that give the illness its name.

The NIMH states that half of bipolar diagnoses occur before the age of twenty-five, so the teenage years are a prime time for first showing symptoms.

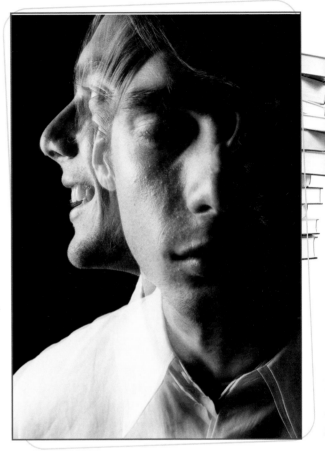

Bipolar disorder brings about extreme shifts in mood between mania and depression, the two poles that give this mental illness its name.

According to the NIMH, about 2.5 percent of teens have bipolar disorder, which is nearly equal to the number of adults (2.6 percent) with the illness. That amount is close to six million people with the disorder in the United States alone.

The Four Types of Bipolar Disorder

The written authority on mental illness is the *Diagnostic and Statistical Manual (DSM)*, which is now in its fifth edition. According to the *DSM-5*, there are four main types of bipolar disorder:

Bipolar I is considered the most severe form, with manic episodes that last at least a week and depression that lasts at least two weeks. The symptoms can be so severe that they require hospitalization.

Bipolar II swings between depression and hypomania, a less intense version of mania. Typically, people with bipolar II experience depression more often than they experience hypomania.

Bipolar not otherwise specified (NOS) is diagnosed when the person doesn't have enough symptoms, or the symptoms do not last long enough for that person to receive a diagnosis of bipolar I or bipolar II.

Cyclothymia is a mild form of bipolar disorder. People with cyclothymia shift back and forth between hypomania and mild depression for a minimum of two years.

If bipolar disorder is left untreated, the symptoms may worsen over time. This progression is why it's important to acknowledge worrisome shifts in your mood so that you can get help *before* a major crisis occurs.

A mixed state occurs when a person feels both deeply depressed and highly irritable or agitated. This state used to be associated only with bipolar I, but the *DSM-5* has expanded the definition to include bipolar II, bipolar-NOS, and even depression alone, which is called unipolar depression. The risk for suicide, already high in those with bipolar disorder, goes up when someone is in a mixed state.

Mania and Hypomania

To be diagnosed with mania, your mood must be euphoric, expansive, or irritable for at least a week—or for any length of time if the symptoms are severe enough to require hospitalization.

An expansive mood is one in which you feel larger than life: energized and creative and certain that the world is just waiting for your next brilliant idea, which is sure to be a huge success. Intense irritability can also be a symptom. This irritability is not the type of irritability where you bark at your sister because she "borrowed" your smartphone. It's feeling as if the tiniest upset will push you over the edge, which can lead to embarrassing—and sometimes dangerous—confrontations.

In mental health speak, periods of time when you have certain symptoms are known as episodes. During a manic episode, a person must show at least three of the following symptoms, four if his or her mood is mostly irritable:

- A decreased need for sleep
- Inflated self-esteem
- More talkative than usual ("pressured speech")
- Thoughts that quickly flit from one idea to another ("racing thoughts")

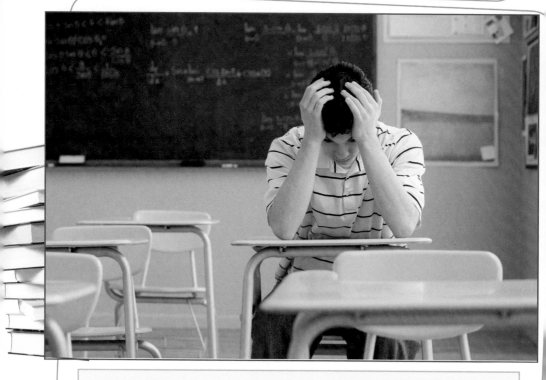

To be diagnosed with mania, your symptoms must have a negative impact on your life in terms of academics, employment, and social functioning.

- Distractibility
- An increase in goal-directed activity
- An increase in sexual behavior
- An inability to keep one's body still ("psychomotor agitation")
- Extreme irritability

As this list suggests, bipolar disorder affects not just mood, but thoughts as well. When in the midst of an episode, it can be difficult to focus or to judge if an idea is brilliant or bound to cause trouble. These symptoms of mania have to have a noticeable negative impact on a person's life in terms of academics, employment, or social functioning. The symptoms can't be related to drug use, medication, or a physical illness.

For the person experiencing mania, some aspects of this mood might sound like fun, but mania can also cause heartache for the person who is ill and everyone around him or her. When manic, you might buy things you can't afford, start projects you can't finish, or get intimately involved with people you shouldn't. Then when the crash comes, you're left cleaning up one gigantic mess.

When hypomanic, a person acts noticeably different from his or her usual self, but the symptoms are less likely to cause long-lasting damage. A person with hypomania will stay up half the night writing a song, while a person with mania will stay up writing the song, then show up at school with her guitar in the morning, insisting on playing that song over the intercom. If her wishes aren't met, she might scream at an administrator, leading to her suspension from school. It's really a matter of degree.

Another difference between mania and hypomania is that with mania there is the possibility of developing psychosis. People with psychosis experience hallucinations—hearing and/or seeing things that aren't real. Delusions are also possible, which means believing bizarre, untrue things about yourself or others. A person who is delusional might believe that he is Jesus, for example, or that his friends are out to do him harm. Psychosis can also be a factor in the most severe forms of depression.

The word "psychosis" is scary, so it's important to remember that just because someone with mania *can* become psychotic doesn't mean that he or she *will* have a psychotic episode. If this psychotic episode does happen, however, there are professionals who can help someone manage this type of disordered thinking.

Depression

The opposite pole of mania is depression. This extreme is what is known as major depression, which is more than just feeling blue after messing up a test or having a fight with your BFF. Major depression sticks around, although the length of each episode differs from person to person. When dealing with major depression, you feel so low that you don't even want to get out of bed, although sleep patterns are often erratic, causing you to sleep too much or too little. The same holds true for food.

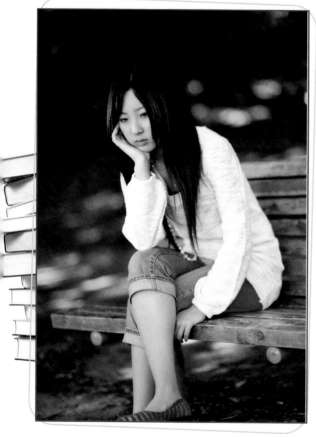

Someone dealing with major depression finds little pleasure in the things that used to bring him or her joy. Sleep and eating patterns also become erratic when a person is depressed.

10

Some in the grips of a major depression have no appetite, while others have the urge to eat everything in sight.

A person going through a major depression loses interest in the people and things that used to bring him or her joy. Your self-esteem takes a hit as you feel both helpless and guilty for not being able to fix your mood. Suicidal thoughts can occur because you just can't imagine slogging through another day feeling so sad and so certain that things will not turn around.

Mood disorders are the psychiatric diagnosis most associated with suicide. The overall number of suicides in the United States is increasing, too. According to the Centers for Disease Control and Prevention (CDC), suicide is the third leading cause of death among children and young people between the ages of ten and twenty-four, behind accidents and homicide. These statistics point to the need for obtaining treatment as early as possible, and the first step in that process is getting a proper diagnosis.

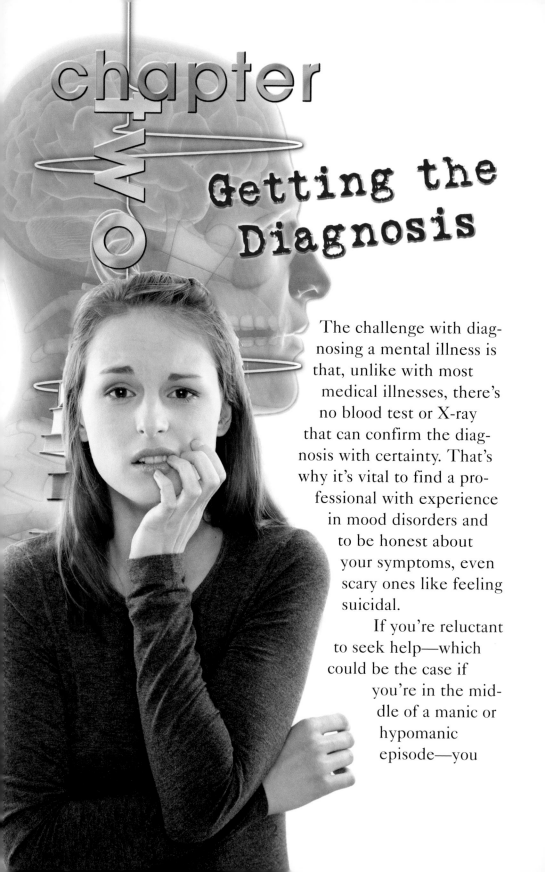

chapter two

Getting the Diagnosis

The challenge with diagnosing a mental illness is that, unlike with most medical illnesses, there's no blood test or X-ray that can confirm the diagnosis with certainty. That's why it's vital to find a professional with experience in mood disorders and to be honest about your symptoms, even scary ones like feeling suicidal.

If you're reluctant to seek help—which could be the case if you're in the middle of a manic or hypomanic episode—you

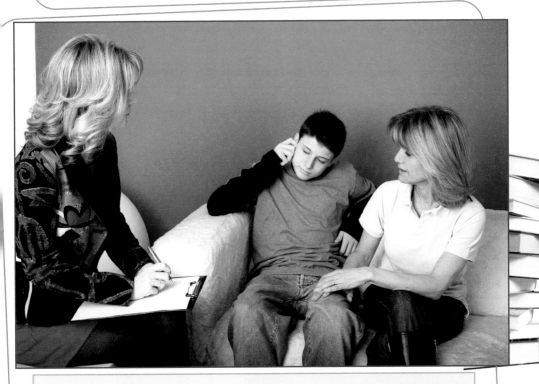

If your parents are reluctant to have you see a mental health professional, ask a school counselor or another trusted adult to help you and your parents talk things through.

need to trust the people who love you when they say that your behavior concerns them. Getting help sooner rather than later is the best way to manage a mood disorder.

If it's your parents who don't want you to see a mental health professional, talk to them about how you're feeling. Odds are that if you're going through a mood episode, there's been some tension in the house already. Perhaps a school counselor or another trusted adult can help you and your parents get a conversation started.

Although it's not ideal, there are some states that allow you to seek counseling without parental permission. That benefit doesn't mean you should stop trying to include your parents in this aspect of your life. Keep the lines of communication open.

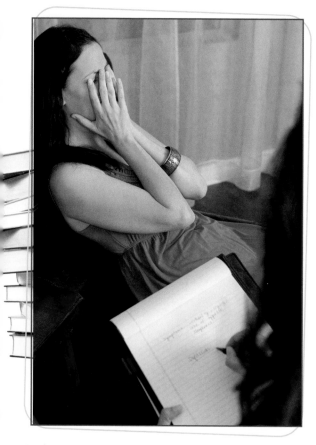

A therapist can help you deal with receiving a diagnosis of bipolar disorder, as well as the lifestyle changes needed to keep your mood steady.

A Team Approach

When setting out to find relief for your shifts in mood and energy, your first stop should be your pediatrician or adolescent medicine doctor. There are physical illnesses that cause symptoms like those of bipolar disorder, so it's important to rule these out before moving on to a specialist in mental health disorders. Conditions that can mimic bipolar disorder include viral infections, autoimmune diseases, thyroid conditions, and hepatitis. Having low levels of vitamin B12, vitamin D, or iron can also affect your emotions and energy.

Once a physical illness has been ruled out, seek the help of a mental health professional trained to deal with mood disorders, such as a psychiatrist, psychologist, or licensed social worker. Psychiatrists are medical doctors and the only providers who can prescribe medications, which are typically an important part of treating bipolar disorder.

Many people with bipolar disorder have more than one professional working with them. This team can include a psychiatrist to prescribe and monitor medications and a therapist to help deal with receiving the diagnosis, as well as the lifestyle changes that bipolar disorder requires.

Whether your initial meeting is with a psychiatrist, psychologist, or social worker, he or she will no doubt have questions to ask about how you've been feeling, including the following:

- What are your symptoms, and how long have you felt this way?
- Have you felt the same way at other points in your life?
- Have you been eating more—or less—lately?
- Has it become more difficult for you to fall asleep or stay asleep?
- Are you struggling in school, either academically or socially?
- Do your moods shift a lot?
- Do you feel more irritable than usual?
- Has anyone pointed out that you seem "not like yourself?"

- How much alcohol do you drink, if any?
- Have you ever experimented with drugs?
- Have you ever felt suicidal, and if so, have you gone so far as to make a plan to kill yourself?

It's never easy to answer personal questions, but you should feel a certain level of comfort with the professional asking you about your mood issues. If you don't, look for someone else to help you. Mental illness is hard enough to handle without feeling as if your psychiatrist or therapist doesn't understand and support you.

Don't forget that you're allowed to ask questions, too. You have the right to know how many years this person has been in practice and how many of his or her patients have bipolar disorder. If he or she believes you have bipolar disorder, ask what led to that conclusion and which particular diagnosis (bipolar I, bipolar II, bipolar-NOS, or cyclothymia) you have.

Dealing with the Diagnosis

If you are diagnosed with bipolar disorder, there's a chance you might also be diagnosed with a second disorder, which is called a co-morbid condition. Attention deficit disorder with or without hyperactivity (ADD or ADHD), generalized anxiety disorder (GAD), eating disorders, and drug and alcohol problems are some of the conditions that can go along with bipolar disorder. The psychiatrist or therapist is not trying to drown you in a sea of diagnoses. Diagnosis does drive treatment, however, so it's important for everyone to know the issues you're facing.

It can be hard to hear that you have bipolar disorder. You might not even believe the therapist or psychiatrist at first, especially if you're manic or hypomanic. If you're severely depressed, the diagnosis gives you yet another reason to feel bad about yourself.

It's OK to be angry when you're told you have a mental illness. Your life will be different from now on, and you will have to make changes to stay well. The most important thing to understand is that you didn't develop bipolar disorder because of your bad behavior or weak will.

Like many other illnesses, a mix of genes and environmental factors cause bipolar disorder. According to Dr. Frances McMahon of the NIMH, when one identical twin has bipolar disorder, the second twin—who shares the first twin's DNA—has a 60 to 80 percent chance of having the disorder as well, showing a strong genetic component. Stressful life events can be an environmental factor in bipolar disorder. Once the disorder is set in motion, however, it seems to take on a life of its own, even after that original stressor has been removed.

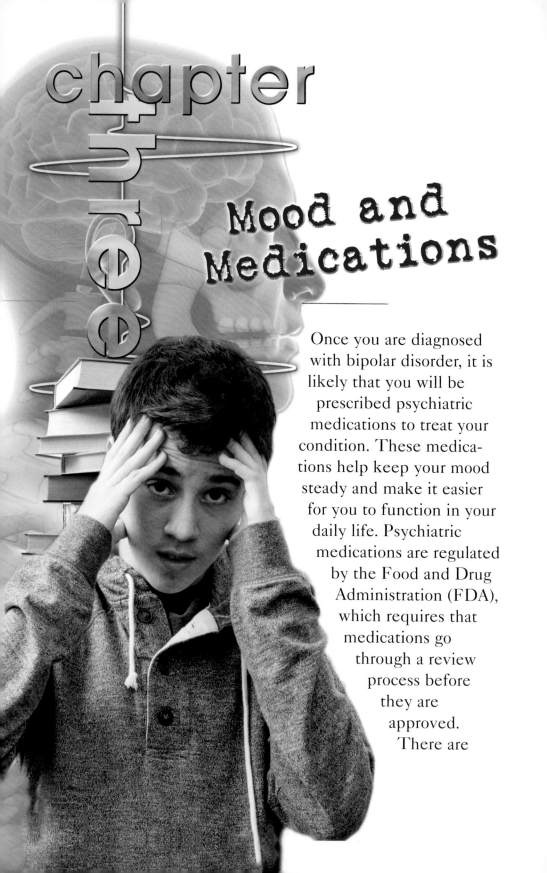

chapter three

Mood and Medications

Once you are diagnosed with bipolar disorder, it is likely that you will be prescribed psychiatric medications to treat your condition. These medications help keep your mood steady and make it easier for you to function in your daily life. Psychiatric medications are regulated by the Food and Drug Administration (FDA), which requires that medications go through a review process before they are approved. There are always new drugs being developed, so the FDA's Web site (www.fda.gov) is a great resource for both patients and doctors.

It can feel frightening to take medications designed to alter your mood, especially knowing that you might have to take them on a long-term basis. It can also take a while to find the right medication, and it's not uncommon to need more than one medication—called a "cocktail" of medications—to help you feel like yourself again.

To manage all this, you need patience and a good relationship with the mental health professionals in charge of your care. It is also important to remember that medications are only *part* of your treatment plan, along with therapy, lifestyle changes, and the help you get from a mental health support group or a twelve-step program for those dealing with drug or alcohol issues.

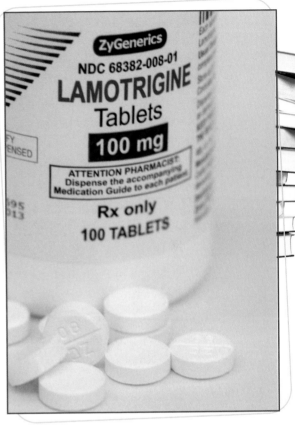

Lamictal, which has the generic name lamotrigine, belongs to a class of medications known as mood stabilizers that can treat the symptoms of bipolar disorder.

Mood Stabilizers

One class of medications widely used to treat bipolar disorder is mood stabilizers. Lithium has been used as a mood stabilizer since the 1960s and works to treat manic episodes and to keep those episodes from coming back. People taking lithium are also less likely to commit suicide. If the dose of lithium is too low, however, the medication won't work, while too high a dose can be toxic. Regular blood tests are needed to make sure that the amount of lithium in your blood stays at a safe but effective level.

Medications designed to treat the neurological disorder epilepsy, which causes surges of electrical activity in the brain called seizures, are also effective as mood stabilizers. As with most drugs, these mood stabilizers have both brand names—those given to them by their manufacturers—and generic names related to their chemical makeup.

The three most common mood stabilizers are Depakote (generic name: valproate), Tegretol (carbamazepine), and Lamictal (lamotrigine). Depakote and Tegretol work well to treat mania, while Lamictal is believed to reduce the number of cycles between mania and depression and to lessen depression in people with bipolar disorder.

These medications do come with a list of possible side effects, including nausea, weight gain, dizziness, liver and pancreas problems, and rare but dangerous skin rashes. Tegretol and Depakote require regular blood tests to make sure you are taking the proper amount without causing any harm to your body. You should never change your dose of any medication without first speaking to the doctor who prescribed it.

Antipsychotics

Antipsychotics are not only used to treat psychosis, although the word might make you think otherwise. They are also useful for treating mania, agitation, and in some cases, depression. Older antipsychotics, known as typical antipsychotics, work well but can cause severe side effects, especially if used for a long time. One of the most worrisome side effects is a neurological disorder called tardive dyskinesia. The symptoms of tardive dyskinesia are involuntary movements such as grimacing, continuous eye blinking, and lip smacking.

Newer antipsychotics are called atypical antipsychotics and are used far more often than typical antipsychotics because, although they are equally effective, they are less likely to cause severe side effects. These medications include Abilify (aripipazole), Geodon (ziprasidone), Risperdal (risperidone), Seroquel (quetiapine), and Zyprexa (olanzapine).

Antidepressants

Although antidepressants can help with depression, they can also lead to manic or hypomanic episodes. For this reason, many psychiatrists are reluctant to put people with bipolar disorder on antidepressants and will only do so after a mood stabilizer is in place. The mood stabilizer might be enough to alleviate the depression and if not, it will help you from becoming manic or hypomanic while taking an antidepressant.

There are many different types of antidepressants, including selective serotonin reuptake inhibiters (SSRIs) such as Prozac (fluoxetine) and Paxil (paroxetine), which are thought to regulate the amount of a neurotransmitter called serotonin in your brain. Other antidepressants include tricyclic antidepressants, which have been in use for more than forty years, and newer drugs such as Effexor (venlafaxine) and Remeron (mirtazapine). If your psychiatrist wants to prescribe an antidepressant, be sure to ask why he or she thinks this medication should be part of your treatment plan, and feel free to voice any concerns you might have about becoming manic while on the drug.

The Best Approach

Every time you turn on the television or flip through a magazine, there seems to be another advertisement for a medication—including psychiatric medications—with another long list of side effects. There are few, if any, benign medications, meaning ones with no possible down-side. The trick is to determine if the rewards of taking a medication are worth whatever side effects you might feel.

Many side effects do lessen over time, so maybe you can tolerate feeling a bit tired or nauseated at first if it means your mood will be more stable. You can try to make adjustments to lessen these effects, as well. If your medications make you feel sleepy, perhaps you can take them at bedtime so that you won't feel like you're in a fog all day. Some drugs can lead to weight gain, so a diet and exercise plan could help, provided that the medication is going a long way toward improving your mood.

There might be times when you don't want to take your medication. The side effects are outweighing the positive effects, or maybe you feel so good that you can't even remember why you needed the medication in the first place. According to the *Psychoeducation Manual for Bipolar Disorder* by Francesc Colom and Eduard Vieta, seven out of ten patients stop taking their medications during their course of treatment.

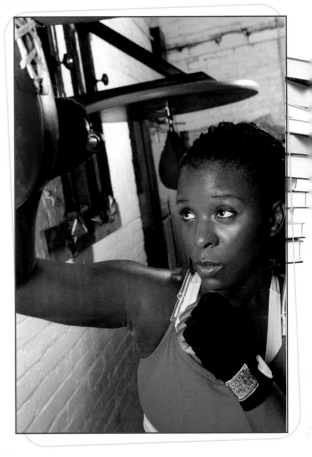

Medications for bipolar disorder can have side effects, including weight gain. A sensible diet and exercise program will help you maintain a healthy weight while on the medication.

Stopping your medications suddenly is risky for both your mind and body. That's why it's so important to have a strong support system in place. You need a psychiatrist who is willing to take the time to find the right medications for you. You also need a therapist and family and friends to help you come to terms with your diagnosis. At times, this might include reminding you of how awful you feel when you're in the middle of a manic, hypomanic, or depressive episode.

MYTHS AND FACTS

Myth: People with bipolar disorder just need a better outlook on life, not medications or therapy.
Fact: It always helps to try to stay positive, but bipolar disorder is a serious illness that requires more than a change in attitude.

Myth: If you have bipolar disorder, you'll never be able to go to college or hold down a job.
Fact: Many people with bipolar disorder can further their education and have a steady job as long as they take care of their mental health and ask for help when it's needed.

Myth: People with bipolar disorder are a danger to society.
Fact: The vast majority of people with mental illness are not dangerous, except perhaps to themselves. In fact, according to the Depression and Bipolar Support Alliance (DBSA) people with mental illness are twice as likely to be *victims* of violence as those without mental illness.

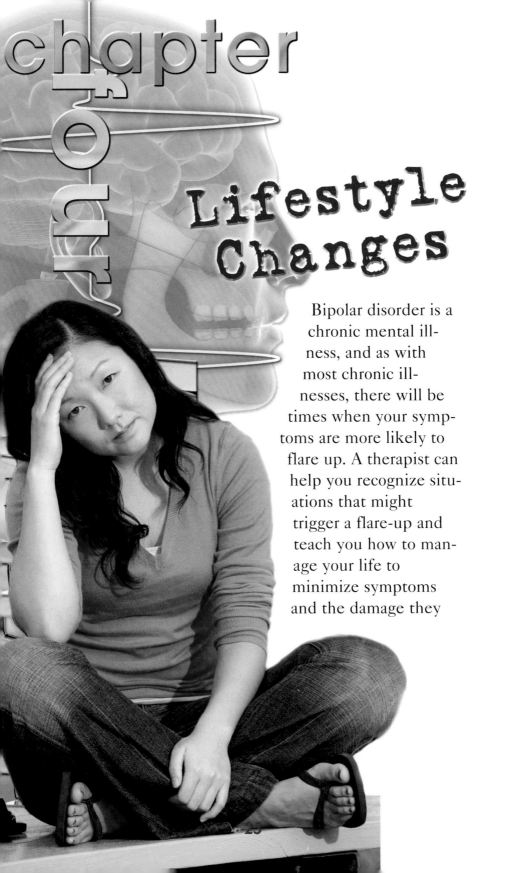

chapter four

Lifestyle Changes

Bipolar disorder is a chronic mental illness, and as with most chronic illnesses, there will be times when your symptoms are more likely to flare up. A therapist can help you recognize situations that might trigger a flare-up and teach you how to manage your life to minimize symptoms and the damage they

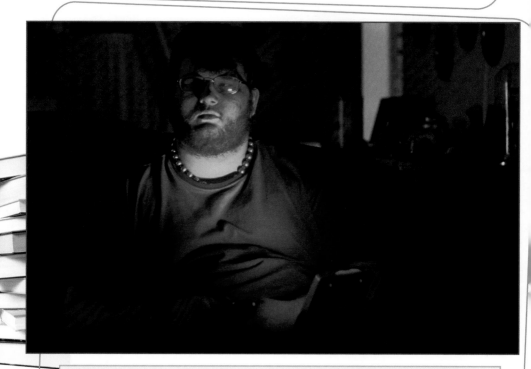

This teen is using light therapy to help with a type of depression known as seasonal affective disorder, which is caused by a lack of light during the winter months.

cause. This type of work is known as psychoeducation and can include not only individual therapy, but also group and family therapy, depending on your needs.

It might help to think of a therapist like a coach, offering tips and strategies to help you handle your illness. The therapist's job is to offer a sympathetic ear and to help you reach your goals on your own terms. Your job is to be honest about the ways in which your illness is affecting your life and any situations that you think might be making things better—or worse.

Structure

In their book *Facing Bipolar: The Young Adult's Guide to Dealing with Bipolar Disorder*, authors Russ Federman and J. Anderson Thomson Jr. talk about the four S's needed to manage bipolar disorder: structure, stress, sleep, and self-monitoring.

Bipolar disorder is an unpredictable illness, so any structure you can add to your life is helpful. Although it might sound like fun to wake up and see where the day takes you, without a routine the day might take you somewhere you shouldn't go. If you're feeling manic or hypomanic, you might spend too much money or get into a fight with a friend. If you're depressed, you might feel like there's no reason to get up at all. Structure is not a miracle cure, but it can help make life seem a little less overwhelming. Adding structure to your life includes doing things such as the following:

- Using a pillbox to organize your medications
- Picking a set time to take your medications every day
- Using a physical or electronic calendar or planner to organize your week
- Eating three balanced meals every day
- Getting to sleep and waking up at the same time each day, even on the weekends
- Getting regular exercise

Some of these ideas seem to go against everything it means to be a teenager, especially getting up early on the weekends! It's true that having bipolar disorder can make you feel as if you're being held back right when you want to be more spontaneous and independent. By following these suggestions, however, you'll be in a better frame of mind to enjoy the hours you do spend at a movie, party, or other activity.

Stress

As a teen, you face a great deal of stress. There's homework to do, your future to think about, and many different kinds of relationships to juggle. Add in the stress of having a mood disorder and the time that doctor visits and therapy sessions require, and you're carrying one heavy load.

People with bipolar disorder need strategies to keep themselves calm, or they risk being flooded with negative thoughts and emotions. One simple technique to lower stress is to focus on taking slow, deep breaths, making sure to inhale through your nose and exhale through your mouth.

It's also important to do things every day to prevent stress from throwing your mood too far off course. You can tailor a program to meet your needs, which is the best way to make sure that you stick with whatever plan you choose. Common stress busters include the following:

- Writing in a journal
- Drawing or painting
- Taking a hot bath
- Listening to music or making music
- Spending time in nature

- Reading
- Talking with a supportive friend or family member

Part of learning how to handle stress is learning to say no to other people. That doesn't mean you should be selfish, just aware of what you need to do to maintain your mental health. There might be days when you don't have an hour to talk to your friend about video games or his latest crush. Depending on how much your friend knows about your illness, you can go into detail or simply ask if you can con-

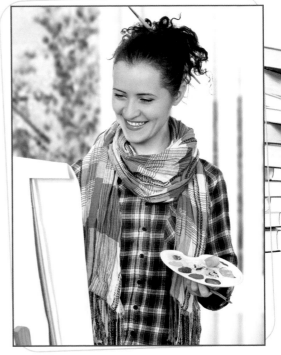

People with bipolar disorder need to keep stress at a manageable level. Activities that can help you deal with stress include listening to music, taking a hot bath, and painting.

tinue the discussion the next day. Of course, if he's in crisis, don't hang up or walk away. The important thing is to recognize that you will never be able to be there for someone else if you don't take care of yourself first.

Sleep

Changes in your sleep pattern can have a huge impact on your mood. If you make a habit of staying up until 1:00 AM to get your homework done, you risk bringing on mania or hypomania. Sleep too much and you might be headed for a depressive episode. Sleeping too much or too little can be a sign that you're *already* in a manic or depressed state, so let your mental health team know about any sleep disturbances. Many things can affect your sleep cycle, including medications and the switch to or from Daylight Savings Time.

Aim for eight or nine hours of uninterrupted sleep per night. Although this might feel restrictive, especially when there's no school the next day, having bipolar disorder means accepting certain changes in your life. Try to focus on how much better you'll feel if you do things that are proven to help steady your mood.

To get a good night's sleep, think of your bed as just that: a place to sleep. It's not a place to watch TV or text your friends or read a book, especially not a thriller that might give you nightmares. Avoid caffeine before bed and try not to take a nap during the day, as this will make it harder to sleep at night. If you're distracted or stressed out by noise, you can listen to recordings of waterfalls or rainstorms or just the hum of white noise. Learn what works for you and try to follow the same steps every time you get ready for bed.

Self-Monitoring

People with bipolar disorder need to keep close track of their mood, thinking, and energy level. In *Facing Bipolar*, authors Russ Federman and J. Anderson Thomson Jr. refer to this as being your own "mood lifeguard." This observation doesn't mean you should spend every waking

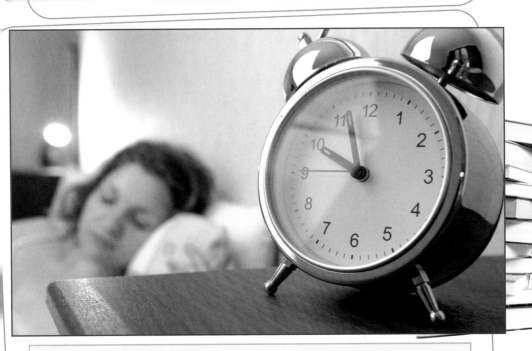

Sleep is vital if you want to keep your mood stable. The goal is to have eight or nine hours of undisturbed sleep per night.

moment worrying whether your mood is up or your energy down, but paying attention to these cues can help head off a more serious episode. There are many resources available to help you do this monitoring in a structured way. The DBSA's Facing Us Clubhouse offers a free wellness tracker, as well as a place to create a personalized wellness plan. There are mood charts available online and even apps you can download if that method suits your style.

You need to have a plan in place should any changes concern you. The plan can include speaking with your psychiatrist about your medications or with your therapist about how your lifestyle might be affecting how you feel. Your parents, school counselor, or another trusted adult can also be a source of support. Make sure you have everyone's contact information with you so that you can reach those most able to help you at a moment's notice.

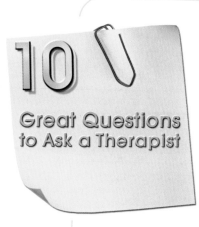

10

Great Questions to Ask a Therapist

1. If there's no medical test for bipolar disorder, how can I be sure I have it?

2. How can I stop feeling like it's my fault that I have bipolar disorder?

3. How do I keep my parents from hovering over me now that I have this diagnosis?

4. Why can't I wait a few years to deal with having bipolar disorder so that I can enjoy being a teenager?

5. How do I avoid feeling resentful toward people who don't have to deal with a mental illness?

6. How do I know that my symptoms are not going to get worse over time?

7. Does having bipolar disorder mean that I shouldn't ever marry or have kids?

8. Where can I meet other teens who are dealing with having a mood disorder?

9. Will there ever be a time I won't need any medication at all?

10. Is anyone ever cured of bipolar disorder?

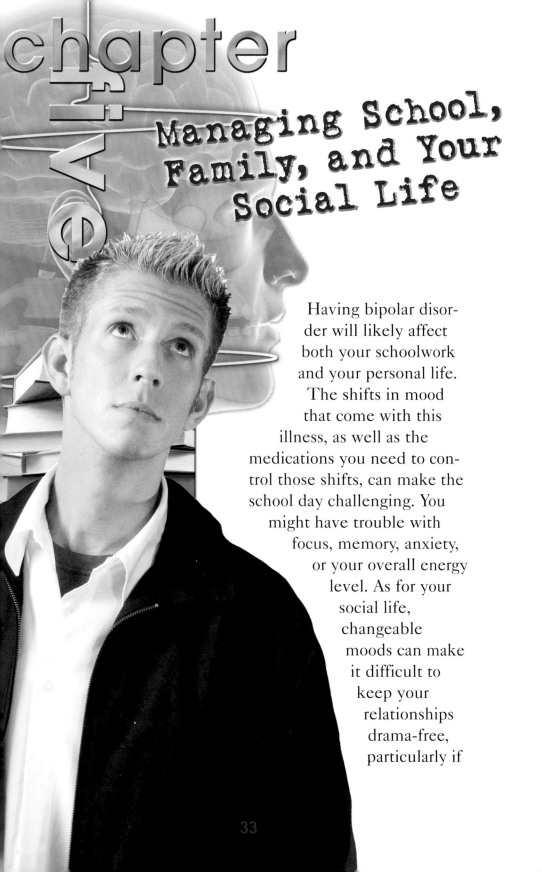

chapter five

Managing School, Family, and Your Social Life

Having bipolar disorder will likely affect both your schoolwork and your personal life. The shifts in mood that come with this illness, as well as the medications you need to control those shifts, can make the school day challenging. You might have trouble with focus, memory, anxiety, or your overall energy level. As for your social life, changeable moods can make it difficult to keep your relationships drama-free, particularly if

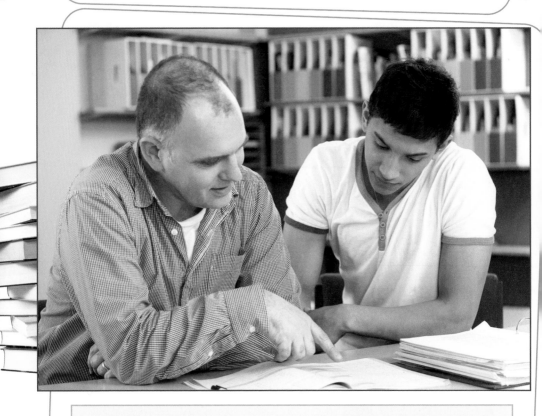

Students with bipolar disorder who are in Individualized Education Programs (IEPs) can receive accommodations such as time in a resource room to go over classwork.

the person you're clashing with doesn't know about your struggles with mental illness. Combine all of this with the need to stick to a routine (which might mean leaving a party early, saying no to sharing junk food, or skipping a sleepover), and it's easy to feel left out. There are ways to work through these problems, however. You just need to be patient and to seek guidance from people who have experience dealing with these issues.

School Success

Students diagnosed with bipolar disorder can be eligible for certain services or modifications—known as accommodations—in their school programs. There are two laws that protect these students, as well as students with other conditions that affect their learning: Section 504 of the Rehabilitation Act of 1973 and the Individuals with Disabilities Education Act (IDEA).

Section 504 offers simple accommodations, such as allowing a student to sit closer to the teacher to help with attention or breaking the lesson down into smaller parts to avoid confusion. Section 504 is usually used for students who spend most of their time in the regular education, or mainstream, classroom.

If you're a student who needs more help than Section 504 offers, services covered by the IDEA might be appropriate. To qualify for these special education services, a student must be tested by a teacher or school psychologist and then placed in one of thirteen classifications. For students with bipolar disorder, the most common classifications are emotionally disturbed and other health impairment. If you qualify, services will be provided through an Individualized Education Program (IEP) that sets out goals for the year and lists the services and accommodations needed to meet those goals. There are a wide range of services and accommodations available, including the following:

- An aide to help with focus, organization, emotional upsets, or other needs

- Time in a resource room to go over work before or after it is presented in a classroom
- Scheduled sessions with the school psychologist
- Scheduled breaks throughout the day
- Extra time for testing
- A later start to the school day when sleep patterns are disrupted

While the law states that it is up to your parents to make educational decisions for you until you reach eighteen, you should encourage them to let you take part in those decisions. Once you reach the point where your "team" (teachers, psychologists, parents, and anyone else involved in your education) starts talking about what you will do once high school ends—called transition—you are *required* to attend IEP meetings.

This whole process can feel overwhelming. You're already dealing with having a mental illness and then you start hearing about testing and IEPs and special education services. It's not enough to have bipolar disorder? You have to be considered disabled? A person who needs special education?

Not everyone with bipolar disorders needs or qualifies for educational services. If you do, however, try to look past the labels and focus on the help you're being offered. Much like your bipolar diagnosis led to proper treatment, Section 504 or an IEP can make your school day far more manageable.

Telling Others About Your Illness

Society is more open-minded about mental illness today than it has been in the past. Many people have dealt with, or know someone who has dealt with, mental health issues. Many celebrities have talked openly about their mood issues, including actress and singer Demi Lovato, who has bipolar disorder. After receiving treatment, Lovato told *People* magazine, "I feel like I am in control now where my whole life I wasn't in control" and stated

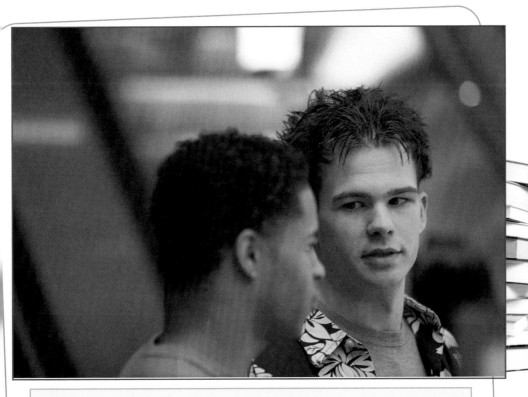

Telling a friend about your bipolar disorder could help him understand your past behavior and bring the two of you closer together.

that her goal was "to help others" struggling with mental illness.

Yet there can still be a stigma attached to mental illness, so caution is needed when talking about your bipolar disorder. You certainly aren't required to tell every person in your life about your illness. Keeping something private is not the same as lying.

If you want to "come out" to someone about having bipolar disorder, think about what might be gained—or lost—by sharing. Telling a friend could help him or her understand why you've behaved the way you have in the past. This friend might be able to point out symptoms to you before those symptoms get out of hand. The two of you might grow closer now that you've shared this part of yourself.

You do risk rejection, however. You always do when you open up to someone. Your friend might be freaked out by your disclosure or afraid of how your illness will affect your relationship. Give your friend time to process this information, but don't set yourself up for more rejection. If you continue to feel shut out, ask yourself how supportive a friendship this has been all along. True friends step up when times get hard and try to understand your concerns, not run away from them.

The same holds true for your dating life. If you have a boyfriend or girlfriend and have done everything possible to keep him or her from seeing you at your worst or knowing about your diagnosis, this is likely an unhealthy relationship. Someone who loves you loves *all* of you, without conditions. A new relationship brings different challenges. You don't need to let someone know about your illness right away, but if the two of you get more serious, you should feel comfortable letting him or her know.

Trust is what's key no matter the situation. If your gut tells you that the other person won't offer support (or will betray you by blabbing to others), keep the information to yourself and take a hard look at the relationship. Having the strength to deal with a difficult diagnosis should earn you *more* respect, not less.

Depending on your situation, your family can be a real source of support or a roadblock. Your parents might hover

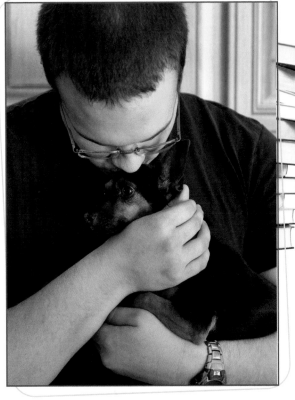

The lifestyle changes that help you manage bipolar disorder, such as lowering stress by spending time with a pet, are healthy habits that everyone should follow.

because they're afraid of letting you out of their sight or they might be deep in denial, leaving you feeling lonely as you face what lies ahead. Try to be honest about what you need from them and remember that no matter how they're acting, they want the best for you.

Having bipolar disorder is not easy, but you should never lose hope based on a diagnosis. A lot of the adjustments it requires will help you lead a healthier life overall. Everyone should try to eat well, get enough sleep, maintain a reasonable routine, learn to reduce stress, and stay attuned to changes in mood and thought.

Although you will likely need medication for your bipolar disorder, you'll have a psychiatrist to help you get the most benefit—and least number of side effects—from any medicine that you take. You'll learn to work with your support system and to open yourself up to new experiences as you continue your journey as a person living—and thriving—with mental illness.

attention-deficit/hyperactivity disorder (ADHD) A disorder that makes it difficult to focus and process information. People with ADHD also have problems sitting still and can be impulsive.

autoimmune disease An illness caused by an overactive immune response to healthy tissue in a person's body.

chronic Going on for a long time or coming back frequently.

diagnosis The process used to determine if a person has a certain mental or physical illness.

euphoric Feeling extremely happy and self-confident; in bipolar disorder, this feeling is exaggerated and unrelated to life events.

genetic Related to the set of traits that a person inherits from his or her parents.

grimacing Twisting of facial expressions to show pain or disgust. In tardive dyskinesia, grimacing is involuntary.

hepatitis A disease that causes inflammation of the liver.

hormones Chemicals released by glands in the body that tell cells to perform certain actions.

navigate To find your way through life's challenges.

prescribed Ordered the use of a certain type of medicine or treatment.

stigma A mark of disgrace given to a person because of a physical or psychological trait or life circumstance.

symptom Something a person feels that indicates a certain illness or disease.

toxic Containing poisonous material that can cause sickness or in some cases, death.

Canadian Mental Health Association (CMNA)
Burnside Building
1110-151 Slater Street
Ottawa, ON K1P 5H3
Canada
Web site: http://www.cmha.ca
The Canadian Mental Health Association is a nationwide organization that provides tools and resources to help people with all types of mental illness lead meaningful and productive lives.

Depression and Bipolar Support Alliance (DBSA)
730 North Franklin Street, Suite 501
Chicago, IL 60610-7224
(800) 826-3632
Web site: http://www.dbsalliance.org
The DBSA provides information on treatment options, mood monitoring, and many other topics related to bipolar disorder.

International Bipolar Foundation
8895 Towne Centre Drive, Suite 105-360
San Diego, CA 92122
(858) 764-2496
Web site: http://www.internationalbipolarfoundation.org
The International Bipolar Foundation is dedicated to advancing research related to bipolar disorder and providing education and support for those with mental health issues.

Juvenile Bipolar Research Foundation (JBRF)
550 Ridgewood Road
Maplewood, NJ 07040
Web site: http://www.jbrf.org
(866) 333-JBRF (5273)
The Juvenile Bipolar Research Foundation focuses on
    research studies and treatments for children and
    teenagers with bipolar disorder.

National Alliance for the Mentally Ill (NAMI)
Colonial Place Three
2107 Wilson Boulevard, Suite 300
Arlington, VA 22201-3042
(800) 950-NAMI (6264)
Web site: http://www.nami.org
The National Alliance for the Mentally Ill offers educa-
    tional programs, discussion groups, and research
    information about bipolar disorder and other mental
    illnesses.

National Federation of Families for Children's Mental Health
9605 Medical Center Drive, Suite 200
Rockville, MD 20850
(240) 403-1907
Web site: http://www.ffcmh.org
This family-run organization focuses on the needs of children
    and youth with emotional, behavioral, or mental
    health issues, as well as their families.

National Institute for Mental Health (NIMH)
Science Writing, Press, and Dissemination Branch
6001 Executive Boulevard, Room 6200, MSC 9663
Bethesda, MD 20892-9663
(866) 615-6464
Web site: http://www.nimh.nih.gov
The NIMH provides information on a wide range of mental illnesses, including resources related to research and advocacy.

Organization for Bipolar Affective Disorders Society
1019-7th Avenue SW
Calgary, AB T2P 1A8
Canada
(403) 263-7408
Web site: http://www.obad.ca
The Organization for Bipolar Affective Disorders offers support and education for those affected by bipolar disorder, depression, and anxiety.

Web Sites

Due to the changing nature of Internet links, Rosen Publishing has developed an online list of Web sites related to the subject of this book. This site is updated regularly. Please use this link to access the list:

http://www.rosenlinks.com/TMH/Bipo

for further reading

Anglada, Tracy. *Intense Minds: Through the Eyes of Young People with Bipolar Disorder.* Murdock, FL: BPChildren, 2009.

Basco, Monica Ramirez. *The Bipolar Workbook: Tips for Controlling Your Moods.* New York, NY: Guilford Press, 2005.

Dougherty, Karla. *Less Than Crazy: Living Fully with Bipolar II.* Boston, MA: Da Capo Press, 2008.

Fieve, Ronald R. *Bipolar Breakthrough.* Emmaus, PA: Rodale Books, 2009.

Fink, Candida, and Joe Kraynak. *Bipolar Disorder for Dummies*, 2nd ed. Hoboken, NJ: John Wiley & Sons, Inc., 2013.

Garey, Juliann. *Too Bright to Hear, Too Loud to See.* New York, NY: Soho Press, 2012.

Simon, Lizzie. *Detour: My Bipolar Road Trip in 4-D.* New York, NY: Washington Square Press, 2003.

Smith, Hilary. *Welcome to the Jungle: Everything You Wanted to Know About Bipolar but Were Too Freaked Out to Ask.* Newburyport, MA: Conari Press, 2010.

Smith, Marybeth. *Fall Girl.* Scotts Valley, CA: CreateSpace Independent Publishing Platform, 2011.

Szabo, Ross, and Melanie Hall. *Behind Happy Faces.* Santa Monica, CA: Volt Press, 2007.

Warner, Judith. *We've Got Issues.* New York, NY: Riverhead, 2010.

Williamson, Wendy K. *I'm Not Crazy, Just Bipolar.* Bloomington, IN: Authorhouse, 2010.

Wilson, Dawn DeAnna. *Saint Jude.* Carraway Bay Press, 2011.

index

A

alcohol and drug use, 9, 16, 19
antidepressants, 21–22
antipsychotics, 21
attention-deficit/hyperactivity
disorder (ADHD), 16

B

bipolar disorder
diagnosis of, 12–17
four types of, 6–7
living with, 25–40
medications, 18–24
myths and facts, 24
what it is, 4–11
bipolar I, 6, 16
bipolar II, 6, 16
bipolar not otherwise specified
(NOS), 6, 16

C

Centers for Disease Control and
Prevention (CDC), 11
co-morbid conditions, 16
cyclothymia, 6, 16

D

depression, 10–11
Depression and Bipolar Support
Alliance (DBSA), 24, 31
Diagnostic and Statistical Manual
(DSM), 6

F

Facing Bipolar, 27, 30
Food and Drug Administration
(FDA), 18, 19

I

Individualized Education
Programs (IEPs), 35–36
Individuals with Disabilities
Education Act (IDEA), 35

M

mania and hypomania, 7–10
medications, 18–24
mood stabilizers, 20–21

N

National Institute of Mental
Health (NIMH), 5, 17

P

psychoeducation, 23, 25–26
Psychoeducation Manual for Bipolar
Disorder, 23

R

Rehabilitation Act of 1973, 35

S

school, success in, 35–36
Section 504, 35, 36

About the Author

Jennifer Landau received her MA degree in creative writing from New York University and her MST in general and special education from Fordham University. An experienced editor, she has also published nonfiction books for young adults. Recent titles include *How to Beat Psychological Bullying* and *Dealing with Bullies, Cliques, and Social Stress.*

Photo Credits